Nursing & Health Survival Guide

Drugs in Use

2nd Edition

Ann Richards

T0033791

R Routledge
Taylor & Francis Group

LONDON AND NEW YORK

First published 2009 by Pearson Education Limited

Second edition 2012

2 Park Square, Milton Park, Abingdon, Oxfordshire OX14 4RN
605 Third Avenue, New York, NY 10017

Routledge is an imprint of the Taylor & Francis Group, an informa business

First issued in paperback 2020

ISBN 13: 978-0-273-76375-8 (pbk)

British Library Cataloguing-in-Publication Data
A catalogue record for this book is available from the British Library

Library of Congress Cataloging-in-Publication Data
A catalog record for this book is available from the Library of Congress

Typeset in 8/9.5pt Helvetica by 35

contents

introduction

Drug administration is an important part of a nurse's role. It is important that the nurse should be able to explain to patients how drugs act and give advice regarding possible side effects and interactions with other medications or diet.

This little book has been designed as a quick reference guide to drugs in common use and their actions. It is not intended as a replacement for more substantial pharmacology texts or for the British National Formulary (BNF). It's designed to be small and accessible so that it can be carried around and referred to easily whilst working in clinical practice.

To achieve these objectives there are sections introducing:

- the general area of pharmacology including mechanisms of drug action
- how the body handles drugs, i.e. absorption, distribution and metabolism
- routes of drug administration
- important classes of drug, e.g. steroids
- drugs used for their action on different body systems, e.g. the respiratory system
- drugs used in some disorders, e.g. diabetes mellitus
- adverse drug reactions
- guidance by the National Institute of Health and Clinical Excellence (NICE) on the use of certain drugs
- features seen in common drug overdoses.

The format makes this little book easy to find your way around and the use of tables enables comparisons to be made between drugs having similar actions, e.g. antiemetics. It is my hope that you will find this guide so informative that it becomes an extremely useful and even indispensable companion as you work with your patients.

Some classes of drugs

Anaesthetic – a drug that renders the patient insensible to stimuli. An anaesthetic may be local, e.g. *lidocaine*, or general, e.g. *propofol*.

Analgesic – a drug that relieves pain. *Morphine* is an example of a very strong analgesic. *Paracetamol* is an example of an analgesic that is available over the counter from chemists.

Anthelmintic – a drug that is used to treat worm infestation, e.g. *piperazine* for the treatment of thread worms.

Antiarrhythmic – a drug used to treat irregularities of heart rhythm, e.g. *amiodarone*.

Antibiotic – antibacterial substance originally derived from fungi or bacteria, e.g. *penicillin*. These drugs are not active against viruses.

Anticoagulant – a drug that inhibits thrombus formation, e.g. *heparin*.

Antidepressant – a drug that helps to relieve depression, e.g. *fluoxetine*.

Antiemetic – a drug that is given to relieve nausea and to stop vomiting, e.g. *metoclopramide*.

Antiepileptic – a drug used to control the seizures in epilepsy, e.g. *sodium valproate*.

Antihistamine – a drug that blocks some action of histamine in the body, e.g. *chlorphenamine*. Histamine is the chemical that is released in hypersensitivity reactions giving the symptoms of hay fever, for example.

Antihypertensive – a drug that reduces blood pressure, e.g. *ramipril*.

Antimicrobial agent – a drug that kills microorganisms, e.g. *vancomycin*.

Antipsychotic – a drug used to treat a psychotic disorder such as schizophrenia, e.g. *haloperidol*. Also known as neuroleptics.

Antipyretic – a drug used to reduce a raised body temperature, e.g. *paracetamol*.

Antiviral – a drug that prevents viruses replicating, e.g. *acyclovir*.

Anxiolytic – a drug that relieves anxiety, e.g. *diazepam*. Such drugs may be dependency producing.

Bronchodilator – a drug that dilates the airways and thus helps breathing, e.g. *salbutamol* (*Ventolin*®) – widely used in treating asthma.

Chemotherapeutic agent – a drug that is selectively toxic to invading microorganisms or tumour cells, e.g. anticancer drugs.

Cytotoxic agent – a drug that kills cells and is used in cancer therapy, e.g. *vincristine*.

Diuretic – a drug that increases urine output, e.g. *furosemide*.

Hypnotic – a drug that induces sleep, e.g. *temazepam*.

Hypoglycaemic agent – a drug that lowers blood glucose, e.g. *metformin*.

Inotrope – a drug that increases the force of cardiac contractions, e.g. *adrenaline*.

Muscle relaxant – a drug that paralyses skeletal muscle, e.g. *atracurium* and is used with general anaesthesia in certain operations.

Vasodilator – a drug that dilates the blood vessels and is sometimes used to bring the blood pressure down, e.g. *amlodipine*.

Common abbreviations used in drug administration

■ LATIN ABBREVIATIONS

ABBREVIATION	MEANING
b.d.	bis die – twice daily
t.d.s.	ter die sumendus – three times daily
t.i.d.	ter in die – three times daily
q.d.s.	quatro die sumendus – four times daily
q.q.h.	quarta quaque hora – every four hours
o.m.	omne mane – every morning
mane	morning
o.n.	omne nocte – every night
nocte	night
p.r.n.	pro re nata – as required
stat	immediately
a.c.	ante cibum – before food
p.c.	post cibum – after food

■ ROUTES OF ADMINISTRATION

ABBREVIATION	MEANING
p.o.	per os – by mouth
n.g.	nasogastric
s.l.	sublingual
IV	intravenous
IM	intramuscular
subcut.	subcutaneous
p.r.	per rectum
p.v.	per vagina
gutt.	eye drops
occ.	eye cream
e/c	enteric coated
m/r	modified release

■ UNITS USED IN DRUG ADMINISTRATION

ABBREVIATION	MEANING
ml	millilitre
l	litre
g	gram
mg	milligram
mcg, μg	microgram
units	International Units

Handy conversions to know

1 g	=	1000 mg
1 mg	=	1000 mcg
1 litre	=	1000 ml

■ RECOGNISED DRUG ABBREVIATIONS

ABBREVIATION	MEANING
ACE	angiotensin-converting enzyme
GTN	glyceryl trinitrate
MAOIs	monoamine oxidase inhibitors
NSAID	non-steroidal anti-inflammatory drug
SSRIs	selective serotonin reuptake inhibitors

■ OTHER COMMON ABBREVIATIONS

ABBREVIATION	MEANING
ADHD	attention deficit hyperactivity disorder
AF	atrial fibrillation
AIDS	acquired immunodeficiency disorder
approx.	approximately
BMI	Body Mass Index
BP	British Pharmacopoeia
CNS	central nervous system
COPD	chronic obtrusive pulmonary disease
CSM	Committee on Safety of Medicines
CVA	cerebrovascular accident

ABBREVIATION	MEANING
CVD	cardiovascular disease
ECG	electrocardiogram
GI	gastrointestinal
HF	heart failure
HIV	human immunodeficiency virus
HRT	hormone replacement therapy
IHD	ischaemic heart disease
INR	international normalised ration
LVF	left ventricular failure
max.	maximum
MHRA	Medicines and Healthcare Products Regulation Agency
MI	myocardial infarction
NHS	National Health Service
NICE	National Institute for Health and Clinical Excellence
NPF	Nurse Prescribers' Formulary
PGD	patient group direction
RTI	reproductive tract infection
UTI	urinary tract infection
VF	ventricular fibrillation
VT	ventricular tachycardia
WHO	World Health Organization
WPW	Wolff-Parkinson-White (syndrome)

Some definitions

Following is a table showing some common terms used in pharmacology.

Pharmacology	The study of the properties of drugs and their effects on the body.
Pharmacist	A person qualified by examination and registered to dispense medicines.
Pharmacodynamics	How drugs affect body cells to produce their action.
Pharmacokinetics	How the body handles a drug. Includes absorption, distribution, metabolism and elimination.
Drug absorption	The passage of a drug into the internal environment of the body.
Drug metabolism	The chemical breakdown of a drug prior to elimination.
Drug elimination	The irreversible movement of the drug out of the body.
Drug excretion	The removal of the products of metabolism from the body.
Bioavailability	The percentage of drug reaching the circulation.
Therapeutic index (TI)	The ratio of the therapeutic dose of the drug to the toxic dose. The higher the TI, the safer the drug.

Plasma half-life ($t_{1/2}$)	Time taken for the plasma level of the drug to decline by half its value.
First pass effect	The metabolism of a drug to an inactive metabolite the first time it passes through the liver.
Pharmacogenetics	The genetic variation that gives rise to individual differences in drug response and metabolism.
Therapeutic drugs	Drugs used for treatment and healing.
Polypharmacy	Treatment of a patient with more than one drug.
Tolerance	Higher doses of the drug become necessary to achieve the same effect.
Dependence	Withdrawal symptoms occur when the drug is stopped.
Prodrug	A drug that needs to be changed by metabolism before it has any action.
Teratogen	A drug that may produce congenital malformation in the unborn child, e.g. *thalidomide*.

Routes of drug administration

A drug may be administered via many routes, the most common of which are orally and intravenously.

ROUTE	EXPLANATION	EXAMPLE
Oral	By mouth as tablets, capsules or as a liquid.	*Paracetamol*
Sublingual or buccal	Under the tongue or between the gum and cheek. The tablet is kept in the mouth and absorbed through mucous membranes into the small blood vessels.	*GTN (glyceryl trinitrate)* for angina
Transdermal	As a patch placed on the skin – the drug is absorbed through the skin for systemic action.	*GTN* for angina *Fentanyl* as analgesia
Topical	Onto a body surface for local action.	Skin creams/ointments
Ocular	Into the eye as drops or ointment.	*Timolol* for glaucoma
Nasally	Into the nose usually as a spray.	*Becotide* for hay fever

ROUTE	EXPLANATION	EXAMPLE
Inhalation	Inhaled into the lungs via a metred dose inhaler or a nebuliser, usually for respiratory tract conditions.	*Salbutamol* for asthma
Rectally	Inserted into the rectum as a suppository or liquid.	Rectal *diazepam* in convulsions
Vaginal	Pessaries and creams inserted into the vagina for local action.	*Nystatin* for thrush
Injections		
Subcutaneous	Under the skin.	*Insulin* in diabetes
Intramuscular	Into a muscle, usually in the thigh.	Occasionally analgesia
Intravenous	Into a vein.	Antibiotics

■ ORAL ADMINISTRATION

ADVANTAGES	DISADVANTAGES
Ease of administration	Has to be absorbed from the gastrointestinal tract
Convenient	Takes time to be absorbed
Non-invasive	Some of the drug may not be absorbed at all
	May be affected by food in the stomach
	Absorption may be unpredictable
	Affected by vomiting or diarrhoea

■ INTRAVENOUS DRUG ADMINISTRATION

ADVANTAGES	DISADVANTAGES
No absorption necessary	Once given cannot be removed
Immediate action	Allergic responses more severe
All drug reaches the bloodstream	Infection is possible – must be aseptic procedure
Rate can be controlled when a continuous infusion is given	Special training needed for administration
	May be uncomfortable

Drug absorption, distribution, metabolism and elimination

■ ABSORPTION

- If a drug is given IV it does not need absorption into the bloodstream but drugs given by all other routes do.
- Oral administration provides the most barriers to drug absorption as there are many membranes for the drug to get through before it reaches the bloodstream.
- Drugs are mostly absorbed by passive diffusion. Absorption is better for:
  - Small molecules
  - Lipid (fat) soluble drugs
  - Uncharged molecules – not ions.

■ DRUG DISTRIBUTION

- Ideally we would like a drug to target the tissue on which we need it to work. This is not usually possible.
- Once a drug is in the bloodstream it is carried all over the body, which explains many of the side effects of drugs.
- Drugs are often transported around the bloodstream attached to plasma proteins.
- Some drugs are concentrated in certain tissues such as adipose tissue or glandular tissue.
- The blood–brain barrier prevents many drugs getting to the brain. Very lipid soluble drugs get through the barrier more easily.

■ DRUG METABOLISM AND ELIMINATION

The rate of elimination of a drug is a major factor in determining its length of action.

- Chemical changes to most drugs occur in the liver using enzymes.
- Stimulation or inhibition of drug-metabolising enzymes can increase/decrease the rate of metabolism of a drug, e.g. alcohol stimulates some liver enzymes.
- If there is liver disease some drugs may accumulate in the body.
- Sometimes the products of metabolism can be toxic, e.g. *paracetamol* in overdose.
- Most drugs are metabolised by the liver and then eliminated in the urine.
- Some drugs are eliminated unchanged in the urine, e.g. *penicillin*.
- Some lipid soluble drugs enter the bile and are eliminated in the faeces.
- Some volatile drugs may be eliminated via the respiratory tract.
- Minor routes of elimination include the skin, breast milk and any bodily secretions.
- It is important to know the means of elimination, as drugs excreted by the kidney would not be given to those with kidney disease.

Mechanisms of drug action – pharmacodynamics

Drugs may work in the following ways:

- Simple chemical action, e.g. an antacid. Combines with and neutralises stomach acid.
- Simple physical action, e.g. an osmotic diuretic such as **manitol**.
- Enzyme inhibition, e.g. **statins** inhibit the rate-limiting enzyme in cholesterol synthesis in the liver.
- Ion channel blockade, e.g. calcium channel blockers such as **amlodipine**.
- Fitting into receptors – most drugs, e.g. **adrenaline**.

Drug receptors

Receptors are proteins on the outside or inside of a cell that bind natural substances such as hormones and neurotransmitters. Many drugs also act by binding to these receptors.

The binding is converted to a signal that the cell understands and responds to in some way, e.g. when adrenaline binds to receptors in the heart muscle, the strength of cardiac contraction increases.

Receptors have the ability to up or down regulate.
If there is a high concentration of the agent that binds to
the receptor, receptors may decrease in number over time.

- **Agonists** are substances that stimulate the receptor and
  bring about a response, e.g. *adrenaline*.
- **Antagonists** bind to a receptor but bring about no
  response. Sometimes these may be known as blockers,
  e.g. beta-blockers such as *atenolol*.

Agonist + receptor → response
Antagonist + receptor → no response

Affinity is the ability of a substance to bind to a receptor.
Efficacy is the ability, once bound, to produce an effect.
Potency is the strength of a drug. A potent drug produces
effects at low concentration.

Some drugs affecting adrenergic transmission

DRUG	MAIN ACTION	SOME CLINICAL USES	UNWANTED EFFECTS	CONTRAINDICATIONS
Noradrenaline	α/β agonist	Acute hypotension	Hypertension, headache, peripheral ischaemia, bradycardia, arrhythmias	Hypertension, pregnancy
Adrenaline	α/β agonist	Cardiac arrest Acute severe asthma Anaphylaxis	Anxiety, tremor, tachycardia, headache, cold extremities In overdosage, arrhythmias, cerebral haemorrhage, pulmonary oedema, nausea, sweating, dizziness	Only cautions such as heart disease and glaucoma

DRUG	MAIN ACTION	SOME CLINICAL USES	UNWANTED EFFECTS	CONTRAINDICATIONS
Dobutamine	β_1 agonist	Cardiogenic shock	Nausea and vomiting, peripheral vasoconstriction, hypotension, hypertension, tachycardia	Tachyarrhythmias, phaeochromocytoma
Salbutamol	β_2 agonist	Asthma and other reversible airway obstruction, premature labour	Fine tremor, headache, muscle cramps, palpitations, tachycardia	Caution in CVD and hypertension
Phenylephrine	α_1 agonist	Acute hypotension Nasal decongestant	Tachycardia, reflex bradycardia, prolonged rise in BP	Cautions as noradrenaline
Dexamfetamine (an amphetamine)	NA release Uptake 1 inhibitor, MAO inhibitor, CNS stimulant	CNS stimulant in narcolepsy ADHD and hyperkinetic states in children Drug of abuse	Hypertension, tachycardia, insomnia, acute psychosis with overdose Dependence	Cardiovascular disease

DRUG	MAIN ACTION	SOME CLINICAL USES	UNWANTED EFFECTS	CONTRAINDICATIONS
Ephedrine	NA release, β agonist	Nasal decongestant	As amphetamine but less	Not given if patient taking MAOIs
Doxazosin	α_1 antagonist	Hypertension, benign prostatic hypertrophy	Postural hypotension, dizziness, weakness, sleep disturbance, tremor	Cautions only
Propranolol	Non-selective β antagonist	Anxiety, migraine, hyperthyroidism	Should not be stopped suddenly especially in IHD, bradycardia, HF, hypotension, heart block, bronchospasm, cold hands and feet, fatigue, nightmares, sexual dysfunction	Asthma, uncontrolled HF, bradycardia, hypotension, heart block

DRUG	MAIN ACTION	SOME CLINICAL USES	UNWANTED EFFECTS	CONTRAINDICATIONS
Atenolol	Selective β_1 antagonist	Angina, hypertension	As propranolol but reduced effects of β_2 blockade – less risk of bronchospasm	As propranolol
Labetolol	α_1/β antagonist	Hypertension in pregnancy, hypertension in anaesthesia, hypertensive crisis	Postural hypotension, bronchoconstriction. See also under propranolol	As propranolol
Carvedilol	α_1/β antagonist	Symptomatic chronic HF, hypertension, angina	Postural hypotension, dizziness. See also propranolol	As propranolol. Avoid in severe HF

Drugs and the respiratory tract

- Main conditions are asthma and COPD.
- Bronchodilators are important in all conditions where bronchospasm and bronchoconstriction occur.
- Drugs often administered via a metred dose inhaler or, in an acute situation, a nebuliser.
- In asthma, steroid inhalers are important as 'preventers'. They do not work immediately but are anti-inflammatory and reduce the number of asthma attacks, preventing chronic changes in the lungs. They must be taken daily, e.g. ***beclometasone***.
- The British Guideline on the management of asthma in adults and children is produced by the British Thoracic Society and takes a stepwise approach. Additional guidelines are also produced for the management of life-threatening asthma.
- NICE produces guidance on the management of COPD in primary and secondary care.

■ BRONCHODILATORS

Bronchodilators are drugs that relax the smooth muscle in the respiratory tract and dilate the airways.

Beta$_2$ agonists
- Stimulate the β_2 (beta$_2$) adrenergic receptors in the airways and antagonise smooth muscle contraction no matter what is causing the spasm. This leads to bronchodilation.
- Inhibit mediator release from mast cells.

- May inhibit vagal tone and increase mucous clearance by an action on the cilia.
- Usually given by inhalation but some available orally and intravenously.

Short acting – *salbutamol (Ventolin®)*, *terbutaline* – taken as needed.
Longer acting – last up to 12 hours – *salmeterol*, *eformotorol*.

Unwanted effects – tachycardia, headache, fine tremor, muscle cramps, palpitations.

Antimuscarinic drugs

IPRATROPIUM (ATROVENT®)

- Blocks the muscarinic acetylcholine receptor (parasympathetic nervous system) and prevents bronchoconstriction due to vagus nerve stimulation.
- Reduces bronchial secretions.
- Given by metred dose inhaler or a nebuliser.
- Used more in COPD.
- May be administered with *salbutamol*.

Unwanted effects – dry mouth, constipation, nausea and headache.

THEOPHYLLINE (AMINOPHYLLINE)

- Bronchodilator used in acute asthma and chronic COPD.
- *Aminophylline* may occasionally be given as an IV infusion in severe acute asthma.
- Slow release may be used in COPD – *Slo-Phyllin*, *Uniphyllin*.

Unwanted effects – general stimulant – tachycardia, nausea, palpitations, insomnia, convulsions. Toxic just above the therapeutic dose.

■ OTHER DRUGS USED IN ASTHMA

Corticosteroids

- Used by inhaler early in asthma when *salbutamol* is being used more than two or three times a week.
- Examples are *beclometasone* (*Becotide*®), budesonide (*Pulmicort*®), fluticasone (*Flixotide*®).
- Extremely important in long-term asthma prevention and treatment.
- Only given orally (as *prednisilone*) in acute, severe asthma.
- Usually only a 5-day course due to side effects.
- Available as *hydrocortisone* to give IV if necessary.

Leukotriene receptor antagonists – *montelukast* (*Singulair*®), zafirlukast (*Accolate*®)

- Block leukotriene receptors.
- Leukotrienes are inflammatory mediators important in some forms of asthma.
- Taken orally in tablet form.

Steroids (glucocorticoids, corticosteroids)

Cortisol is produced by the adrenal gland.
   Function in health is to combat stress.

- Increase blood glucose by protein and carbohydrate breakdown.
- Redistribute body fat – 'moon face', 'buffalo hump'.
- Powerful anti-inflammatory and immunosuppressive action.

Uses

Replacement if not enough steroids produced.

Anti-inflammatory and immunosuppressive uses include:

- Auto-immune diseases, e.g. rheumatoid arthritis
- Hypersensitivity diseases, e.g. asthma, hay fever, eczema
- Inflammatory bowel disease – ulcerative colitis, Crohn's disease
- Prevention of transplant rejection
- Some cancers, e.g. leukaemia, Hodgkin's disease
- Local inflammatory conditions in the eye, ear, nose, skin, etc.
- Smallest dose possible used and systemic use avoided if possible
- Steroid card must be carried as need extra if in stressful situation, e.g. operation, trauma

ROUTE OF ADMINISTRATION	EXAMPLE DRUGS	USES
Parenteral – IV, IM	Hydrocortisone Dexamthasone	Acute adrenal insufficiency To replace oral therapy, e.g. in operations Cerebral oedema
Oral	Hydrocortisone Prednisilone	Replacement therapy As anti-inflammatory or immunosuppressant in disease. Often as short course in severe asthma

ROUTE OF ADMINISTRATION	EXAMPLE DRUGS	USES
Metred dose inhaler	Beclometasone Fluticasone Budesonide	Important in asthma treatment as a preventer of attacks
Nasal spray	Beclometasone (Beconase®)	Allergic rhinitis including hay fever
Eye drops	Betamethasone	Inflammatory eye conditions under expert advice
Skin cream or ointment Different potencies available	Hydrocortisone Betamethasone (Betnovate®)	Eczema, contact dermatitis, insect stings and other skin conditions not due to infection
Rectally as enema	Prednisilone	Ulcerative colitis

Unwanted effects

Increase with increased dosage. Exaggeration of normal effects of steroids occurs.

- If given systemically for a period over three weeks adrenal suppression occurs and need to be withdrawn slowly.
- Hypertension and fluid retention.
- Muscle wasting, fat redistribution, diabetes mellitus.
- Osteoporosis and fractures with long-term use.
- Increased susceptibility to and severity of infections.
- Occasional psychiatric reactions, e.g. euphoria, nightmares, insomnia, mood swings.

Cardiovascular drugs

■ NITRATES

- Vasodilators – affect both the venous system and the arterial systems.
- Converted to nitric oxide in the blood vessels and this relaxes smooth muscle.
- Venous capacitance is increased, reducing venous return and preload on the heart.
- Dilation of arteries reduces peripheral vascular resistance and makes cardiac contraction easier, thus improving cardiac output and reducing the work of the left ventricle.
- Cannot dilate arteries diseased with atheroma but can dilate cardiac collateral circulation.

Uses

- Rapid symptom relief in stable angina – *glyceryl trinitrate* (GTN) given sublingually as a tablet or buccally as a spray – lasts 20–30 min. Not effective orally due to high first pass effect.
- GTN available as patches applied to the skin and worn during the daytime to prevent angina.
- *Isosorbide mononitrate* and *dinitrate* (ISMN, ISDN) given orally as prophylaxis for angina.
- Nitrates available as an IV infusion for use in severe ischaemia and MI.
- Acute LVF – decrease preload and afterload thus lessening the work to be done by the heart.

Unwanted effects include postural hypotension, flushing and headache.

Tolerance occurs if nitrates given continuously. Need a nitrate-free period of about 8 hours in every 24 hours.

■ CALCIUM CHANNEL BLOCKERS

- Interfere with passage of calcium through cell membranes.
- Calcium is needed for smooth muscle contraction, so they relax smooth muscle and thus vasodilate.
- Some also reduce cardiac contractility.
- Dihydropyridine group (non-rate limiting) includes *amlodipine*, *felodipine*, *isradipine*, *nifedipine* and *nimodipine*. These drugs least affect cardiac contractility and rate.
- *Diltiazem* and *verapamil* reduce cardiac contractility and are NOT given in HF or with a beta-blocker.

Uses

- Angina prophylaxis.
- Hypertension.
- *Verapamil* is antiarrhythmic and occasionally used in SVT. Reduces cardiac output and slows the heart rate. May precipitate HF.

Unwanted effects include headache, flushing, oedema, fatigue, palpitations, constipation.

■ ALPHA ADRENORECEPTOR ANTAGONISTS

Block the adrenergic α_1 (alpha$_1$) receptors present on peripheral blood vessels. Stimulation of these receptors by noradrenaline causes vasoconstriction so blockade leads to vasodilation.

Prazosin, doxazosin, indoramin, terazosin

Uses
- Hypertension.
- Cardiac failure.
- Benign enlarged prostate (relax smooth muscle in prostate and improve flow of urine).

Unwanted effects include dizziness, profound hypotension (especially if taking diuretics), headache, tachycardia.

■ POTASSIUM CHANNEL ACTIVATORS

Nicorandil – also has a nitrate component and is used in angina.

■ ACE-INHIBITORS

Captopril, cilazapril, enalapril, fosinopril, imidapril, lisinopril, moexipril, perindopril, quinapril, ramipril, trandolapril
- Renin, released by the kidney, converts angiotensinogen (produced in the liver) into angiotensin I.
- Angiotensin I is converted to angiotensin II by angiotensin converting enzyme (ACE).
- Angiotensin II is a powerful vasoconstrictor and raises blood pressure (BP).
- Angiotensin II also increases the release of aldosterone from the adrenal cortex. This leads to sodium and water retention, thus raising BP, and potassium loss.
- ACE-inhibitors inhibit the enzyme ACE and so prevent the formation of angiotensin II by this route.

- Vasoconstriction does not occur – but vasodilation does.
- Sodium and water are not retained and some diuresis occurs. Potassium is retained.

Uses
- Hypertension. May reduce BP rapidly – first dose is taken at bedtime.
- Used for hypertension in diabetes as they may reduce nephropathy (kidney damage).
- Heart failure – reduce preload and afterload. Increase longevity and decrease symptoms.
- Following MI to prevent further CVD and stroke.

Unwanted effects and cautions
- First dose hypotension especially if already taking a diuretic.
- Potassium retention. May be good if taking a diuretic such as *furosemide* but can lead to hyperkalaemia if not.
- Not given in severe renal stenosis as they may cause renal failure.
- Need to check renal function, urea and electrolytes before starting and monitor.
- Persistent dry cough may occur.

■ ANGIOTENSIN-II RECEPTOR ANTAGONISTS

Candesartan, eprosartan, irbesartan, losartan, olmesartan, telmisartan, valsartan

- Block the receptors for angiotensin II and thus vasodilate and have a small diuretic effect like ACE-inhibitors.
- Do not block ACE and so do not have the side effect of a dry cough.
- Used when patient cannot take ACE-inhibitors.

Drugs affecting cardiac contractility

■ DIGOXIN

- Increases the force of cardiac contraction (positive inotrope).
- Reduces heart rate by decreasing conductivity in the atrioventricular (AV) node.
- Has a long half life and only administered once daily.

Uses

- Atrial fibrillation (AF) to slow ventricular rate.
- Heart failure, especially if AF is present.

Unwanted effects

Adverse effects are dose related and may be signs of digoxin toxicity. Therapeutic dose is close to the toxic dose and levels can be monitored.

- Non-cardiac effects include anorexia, nausea, vomiting and diarrhoea.
- Visual disturbances – blurring, colour vision changes, photophobia.
- Cardiac arrhythmias such as extra beats or heart block.
- Side effects more likely if potassium levels are low (hypokalaemia) or there are other electrolyte disturbances. Also in hypoxia and acidosis.
- Dose may be omitted if pulse rate is below 60.

■ ADRENALINE

- Stimulates all adrenergic receptors.
- Increases the force of cardiac contraction thus increasing cardiac output.
- Relaxes smooth muscle in respiratory tract, causing bronchodilation.
- Vasoconstricts arterioles thus increasing blood pressure.

Uses

- **Cardiac arrest** – administered via a central line at a concentration of 1 in 10 000 (100 micrograms per ml). 10 ml are given (see resuscitation guidelines at www.resus.org.uk).
- **Anaphylaxis** – administered IM – 0.5 mg of adrenaline 1 in 1000, i.e. 0.5 ml.
- **Acute severe asthma** that does not respond to salbutamol.

■ ATROPINE

Antimuscarinic, i.e. blocks the muscarinic acetylcholine receptor and decreases the activity of the parasympathetic nervous system.

- Increases heart rate and may be used to treat bradycardia especially with hypotension and following MI.
- Decreases smooth muscle contraction in the GI tract so may be used to relieve muscle spasm here.
- Decreases bronchial secretions and laryngeal or bronchospasm due to vagal stimulation. May be used in theatre for this purpose.
- Dilates the pupil of the eye and available as eye drops.

■ BETA-ADRENERGIC ANTAGONISTS (BETA-BLOCKERS)

Block the β adrenergic receptor for noradrenaline and adrenaline.

- Two main subtypes of beta receptor – β_1 (mainly in the heart) and β_2 (in the airways, peripheral blood vessels and many other organs).
- Stimulation of β_1 receptors increases force of cardiac contraction and the rate.
- Beta-blockers decrease the force of cardiac contraction (negative inotropes) and slow heart rate.

Uses

- Prophylaxis in angina and post MI – some, e.g. *atenolol*, are cardioselective.
- Hypertension, e.g. *atenolol*.
- Antiarrhythmics, e.g. *esmolol*, *sotalol*.
- Used by specialists in stable chronic heart failure, e.g. *bisoprolol*, *carvediliol*.
- Anxiety and hyperthyroidism, e.g. *propranolol*.
- As eye drops in glaucoma, e.g. *timolol*.
- Prophylaxis of migraine, e.g. *propranolol*.

Unwanted effects

- Bronchoconstriction in asthma – may be life-threatening and are not prescribed to asthmatics.
- May precipitate heart failure in certain circumstances.
- Sleep disturbances and depression occasionally.
- Peripheral vasoconstriction.
- Should be withdrawn slowly.

Antiarrhythmic drugs

All drugs used to treat arrhythmias can also cause them and these drugs are only used by specialists following precise diagnosis of the arrhythmia.

May be classified according to effect on conduction (Vaughan Williams) or, more usefully, according to their clinical use.

■ VAUGHAN WILLIAMS CLASSIFICATION OF ANTIDYSRHYTHMIC DRUGS

CLASS	MECHANISM OF ACTION	EXAMPLES
I	Membrane stabilisation by sodium channel blockade	Lidocaine Flecainide
II	Beta adrenergic blockade	Esmolol
III	Increase refractory period by repolarising K^+ currents	Amiodarone Sotalol
IV	Calcium channel blockade	Verapamil
IV-like	K^+ channel opener	Adenosine

■ EXAMPLES OF DRUGS USED FOR SPECIFIC CARDIAC ARRHYTHMIAS

ARRHYTHMIA	DRUG	USES
Drugs only used in supraventricular arrhythmias	Adenosine*	Paroxysmal SVT + in WPW
	Verapamil	SVT – not WPW
	Esmolol	Control of ventricular rate
	Digoxin	Slows ventricular response in AF
Drugs used in ventricular arrhythmias	Lidocaine* Flecainide Amiodarone*	Ventricular arrhythmias including VT, especially after MI Nodal and ventricular tachycardias, VF
Drugs used in supraventricular and ventricular arrhythmias	Amiodarone* Beta-blockers Dispopyramide Flecainide	As above + SVT, AF and flutter

* most frequently used

Magnesium

- Used intravenously for certain serious arrhythmias including a special type of ventricular tachycardia known as *torsades de pointes*.
- Also may prevent recurrent seizures in eclampsia.
- Used to treat life-threatening asthma when other drugs are not effective.

Lipid-lowering drugs

Raised levels of LDL cholesterol are important in the formation of atheroma in the arteries and are a risk factor for CVD.

■ STATINS

Atorvastatin, fluvastatin, pravastatin, rosuvastatin, simvastatin

- Most important drugs to lower cholesterol.
- Inhibit an enzyme in the liver that is needed for the synthesis of cholesterol.
- Reduce the incidence of CVD.
- Prescribed to all those at risk, especially those with diabetes.

Unwanted effects

- Contraindicated in liver disease.
- Muscle effects – aching and myositis. May cause breakdown of muscle and should be stopped if creatinine kinase levels are raised.
- Patients should report any muscle pain.

■ FIBRATES

Bezafibrate, ciprofibrate, fenofibrate, gemfibrozil

- Mainly decrease triglyceride levels.
- Less effect on LDL cholesterol levels.
- Prescribed if triglycerides raised – risk factor in CVD.

NICE guidance to choice of drug treatment for newly diagnosed hypertension

Start at step 1 and then add on drugs if BP not controlled.

A = ACE-inhibitor (e.g. *ramipril*)

C = Calcium channel blocker (e.g. *amlodipine*)

D = Diuretic (thiazide, e.g. *chlortalidone, indapamide, bendroflumethiazide*)

Step 1
- Younger than 55 years – **A**.
- Older than 55 years or black patients (African or Caribbean descent) of any age – **C**.

Step 2
A + C

Step 3
A + C + D

Step 4 Resistant hypertension
A + C + D + consider further diuretic therapy, e.g. *spironalctone* or alpha-blocker, e.g. *doxazosin* or beta-blocker, e.g. *atenolol*.
Consider seeking expert advice.

Prevention of CVD

- Diet and lifestyle most important.
- **Aspirin** and **statins** are prescribed according to the percentage risk of developing CVD over the next 10 years. Risk tables printed in the BNF.
- Hypertension should be controlled.

Secondary prevention of myocardial infarction

Following an MI, NICE recommends a combination of:
- ACE-inhibitor
- Antiplatelets – usually *aspirin* and/or *clopidogrel*
- Beta-blocker
- Statin

Chronic heart failure

Drugs used to treat CHF include:
- Diuretics – usually *furosemide*
- ACE-inhibitors or angiotensin II receptor blockers (ARBs)
- *Hydralazine* (a vasodilator drug) in combination with *nitrates* if intolerant of ACE-inhibitors and ARBs
- Beta-blockers – reduce the effects of stimulation of the sympathetic nervous system
- *Spironolactone* – an aldosterone antagonist
- *Digoxin* – usually if atrial fibrillation is present

Antithrombotics

The treatment and prevention of thrombosis involves three classes of drugs:

- Anticoagulants
- Antiplatelet drugs
- Fibrinolytics

■ ANTICOAGULANTS

Anticoagulants inhibit the clotting cascade.

Uses

Prevent thrombus formation or extension of an existing thrombus.

HEPARIN

- Heparin inhibits blood clotting by stopping the formation of fibrin.
- Binds to antithrombin III and potentiates its inhibitory action.
- Not absorbed from the gastrointestinal tract and has to be given by injection.
- Intramuscular injection **must not be used** as it causes haematomas.
- Heparin action is immediate.

LOW MOLECULAR WEIGHT HEPARINS (LMWH)

Bemiparin sodium (Zibor®), dalteparin sodium (Fragmin®), enoxaparin sodium (Clexane®), reviparin sodium (Clivarine®), tinzaparin sodium (Innohep®)

- Longer duration of action than standard or unfractionated heparin.
- May be given once daily by subcutaneous injection.
- More predictable response.
- Do not need to monitor using blood tests.

Unwanted effects of heparin

Haemorrhage, skin necrosis, thrombocytopaenia (low platelet count), hyperkalaemia (high potassium level), hypersensitivity reactions (including urticaria, angioedema, and anaphylaxis), osteoporosis after long use.

Contraindications

Haemophilia and other haemorrhagic disorders, thrombocytopaenia, peptic ulcer, recent cerebral haemorrhage, severe hypertension, severe liver disease, following major trauma or recent surgery, hypersensitivity to heparin.

Oral anticoagulants

WARFARIN

Prevents the reduction of Vitamin K which is needed for the clotting process.

Antidote for warfarin is Vitamin K.

- Interferes with the formation of Vitamin K-dependent clotting factors (Factors II, VII, IX and X).
- Delay in onset of action is 2–7 days as clotting factors present in the blood have to be degraded before the warfarin will have an effect.
- **Oral warfarin** is absorbed quickly and totally from the gastrointestinal tract.
- **Action is monitored** by its effect on the **prothrombin time (INR measured)**.
- Considerable variability in warfarin's effect on patients. Effectiveness influenced by age, racial background, diet and other drugs.

Unwanted effects

- Mainly **haemorrhage** – GI tract, urinary tract, soft tissues, oropharynx, intracranial.
- Risk of bleeding highest at start of treatment.
- Crosses the placenta and not given in first months of pregnancy – teratogenic.
- Hypersensitivity and skin rashes, alopecia, purpura.

Examples of drug interactions with warfarin

Reduced protein binding (increased action)	Reduced absorption of Vitamin K
Aspirin	Broad spectrum antibiotics
Sulfinpyrazone	Laxatives
Chlorpromazine	
Inhibition of metabolism of warfarin	**Enhanced metabolism of warfarin**
Cimetidine	Phenytoin
Erythromycin	Barbiturates
Sodium valproate	Carbamazepine
Cranberry juice	St John's Wort
Reduced synthesis of clotting factors	**Enhanced risk of peptic ulceration**
Phenytoin	Aspirin
Salicylates	NSAIDs, corticosteroids
Thrombolytics	**Antiplatelet drugs**
Streptokinase	Aspirin
Tissue plasminogen activator	NSAIDs

New oral anticoagulants

At present recommended by NICE for thrombus prevention following hip and knee replacements.

Dabigatrin

- A direct thrombin inhibitor.
- Rapid action and does not require monitoring when established.
- Most common side effect is bleeding.

Rivaroxaban

- Direct inhibitor of activated clotting factor Xa.
- Does not require monitoring when established.
- Main side effects are nausea and bleeding.

■ ANTIPLATELET DRUGS

Reduce the ability of platelets to stick together. Important in secondary prevention of CHD – **75 mg of aspirin daily** is recommended by NICE.

- **Aspirin** irreversibly inhibits the enzyme *cyclo-oxygenase* (COX). This enzyme is found in platelets and needed for the manufacture of a prostaglandin needed for adherence.

ADP (adenosine diphosphate) is used by platelets to help adherence.

- **Dipyridamole** inhibits an enzyme needed for the use of ADP.
- **Clopidogrel** irreversibly blocks ADP receptors on the platelet surface.

■ THROMBOLYTIC AGENTS

Used in myocardial infarction if emergency angiography not possible and sometimes thrombotic stroke to break up an existing thrombus by helping pathways that are involved in clot breakdown or mimicking molecules such as tissue plasminogen activator (tPA).

Streptokinase, alteplase, tenecteplase, reteplase

- Main adverse effect is bleeding.
- **Hypersensitivity**, especially with *streptokinase* – flushing, breathlessness, rash, urticaria and hypotension. Severe anaphylaxis is rare.

Contraindications to thrombolysis

ABSOLUTE	RELATIVE
Recent or recurrent haemorrhage, trauma or surgery, coagulation defects Active peptic ulceration Oesophageal varices Coma, recent or disabling CVA Hypertension, aortic dissection	Previous peptic ulceration Warfarin Liver disease Heavy vaginal bleeding

Diuretics

Drugs that increase urine output.

Uses

- To reduce oedema in:
  - heart failure
  - renal disease
  - cirrhosis of the liver
  - acute pulmonary oedema
- Hypertension
- Cerebral oedema (***mannitol***)

Unwanted effects

- Dehydration, especially in the elderly.
- Electrolyte imbalance – loss of potassium (unless potassium sparing).
- Sodium and magnesium loss.
- Calcium may be lost (e.g. ***furosemide***) or retained (e.g. ***thiazides***).

SOME COMMON DIURETICS

DIURETIC	SITE OF ACTION	SPECIAL FEATURES	SIDE EFFECTS
Loop diuretics, e.g. *furosemide, bumetanide*	Ascending limb of loop of Henle	Most potent diuretics High ceiling – increased dose produces increased diuresis Venodilator – useful in acute LVF Available orally and IV	Potassium (K) loss a problem with repeated use – may be combined with K-sparing diuretic Deafness with large doses (furosemide) Dehydration if intake not good Magnesium, sodium and calcium loss Hypotension
Thiazides, e.g. *bendroflumethiazide chloralidone, inapamide, metolazone*	Early part of distal tubule	Used as antihypertensives as well as diuretics Have some vasodilatory action Less potent as diuretics than loop diuretics	Potassium loss not a problem with small doses used in hypertension but important in higher doses Low magnesium levels Gout

DIURETIC	SITE OF ACTION	SPECIAL FEATURES	SIDE EFFECTS
Potassium-sparing diuretics, e.g. *amiloride*	Distal tubule	Conserve potassium so used with other diuretics for this purpose	Hyperkalaemia may be a problem if used on own. Should not be used with potassium supplements. Extra caution with ACE-inhibitors
Aldosterone antagonist, e.g. *spironolactone* *eplerenone*	Inhibits action of aldosterone on distal tubule	Potassium sparing and has weak diuretic action Used in CHF and liver disease	Hyperkalaemia No potassium supplements and care with ACE-inhibitors Gynaecomastia with *spironolactone*
Osmotic diuretics, e.g. *mannitol*	Tubular fluid	Increase osmolarity Used to relieve cerebral oedema Given by rapid IV infusion	Chills, fever

Urinary incontinence

This is involuntary urination.

Could be stress incontinence, urge incontinence or overflow incontinence.

Stress incontinence – due to sphincter being inefficient.
Treatment:
- Pelvic floor exercises.
- *Duloxetine* increases sphincter tone. It is a noradrenaline and serotonin reuptake inhibitor.

Urge incontinence – usually due to detrusor (bladder muscle) instability.
Treatment:
- Bladder retraining.
- Severe case antimuscarinic drugs used, e.g. *flavoxate*, *oxybutinin*, *propiverine*, *tolteridone*.
- Caution in heart disease and elderly as may exacerbate CHF.

Overflow incontinence – mainly men with prostate enlargement.
Treatment:
- Alpha-adrenergic blocking drugs are used, e.g. *tamsulosin*.
- Relaxes smooth muscle but lowers blood pressure.
- Antiandrogen *finasteride* may also be used to treat prostatic enlargement.

Gastrointestinal tract

Antacids

- Symptomatic relief of dyspepsia due to reflux oesophagitis, gastritis, hiatus hernia or peptic ulcers.
- Bases that neutralise stomach acid (pH 1–2).
- Given when symptoms are present.

Drugs that decrease acid secretion in the stomach

- Histamine (H_2) antagonists, e.g. ***ranitidine, famotidine*** – reduce acid secretion in peptic ulcer disease or reflux oesophagitis. Allow the ulcer to heal.
- Proton pump inhibitors, e.g. ***lansoprazole, omeprazole*** – more effective to reduce acid secretion. Used to prevent ulcers when NSAIDs are prescribed. Also used with antibiotics to treat peptic ulcers due to *Helicobacter pylori*.

Antispasmodics

- Relax the smooth muscle in the intestines.
- Useful in irritable bowel syndrome and diverticular disease.

DRUG NAME	EXAMPLE	SPECIAL FEATURES
Antacids		
Aluminium salts	Aluminium hydroxide	Tends to constipate
Magnesium salts	Magnesium trisilicate	Tends to be laxative

DRUG NAME	EXAMPLE	SPECIAL FEATURES
Combinations	Aluminium and magnesium salts	Reduces colonic side effects
Alginates added	Gaviscon®	Form layer on top of gastric contents and reduce reflux
Antifoaming agent – simeticone	Infacol® Maalox Plus®	Relieves flatulence and hiccups
Decrease acid secretion		
Proton pump inhibitors	Lansoprazole, omeprazole, pantoprazole	May mask symptoms of stomach cancer
H_2-receptor antagonists	Ranitidine, Famotidine, Nizatidine	May mask symptoms of stomach cancer
Antispasmodics		
Antimuscarinics	Dicloverine (Merbentyl®) Hyoscine (Buscopan®)	Block parasympathetic activity that increases smooth muscle contraction
Direct muscle relaxants	Mebeverine (Colofac®) Peppermint oil	May relieve pain in irritable bowel syndrome

DRUG NAME	EXAMPLE	SPECIAL FEATURES
Antimotility		
Opioids	Codeine phosphate	Also a cough suppressant
Co-phenotrope	Lomotil®	Used in uncomplicated diarrhoea
Loperamide	Imodium®	Used in uncomplicated diarrhoea
Laxatives		
Bulk forming. Best to increase fibre in diet if possible.	Ipaghula (Fybogel®) Methyl cellulose (Celevac®) Sterculia (Normacol®)	Increase faecal mass and so stimulate peristalsis. Also useful in stoma patients and ulcerative colitis
Stimulant laxatives	Bisacodyl (Dulcolax®) Senna (Senokot®) Dantron (Co-danthromer®) Sodium picosulfate	Increase intestinal motility and may cause cramps Used in terminally ill Used prior to bowel surgery
Faecal softeners	Liquid paraffin Arachis oil	Avoid prolonged use As enema in management of haemorrhoids and anal fissure

DRUG NAME	EXAMPLE	SPECIAL FEATURES
Osmotic laxatives	Lactulose Magnesium (Mg) salts	Increase water in the bowel Rapid bowel evacuation with Mg
Bowel cleansing	Citramag®, Klean-Prep®, Moviprep®, Picolax®	Used before colonic surgery, colonoscopy or other investigations. Not used to treat constipation

Antiemetics

Drugs used to prevent and treat nausea and vomiting due to different causes.

The vomiting centre in the brainstem and the associated chemoreceptor trigger zone (CTZ) in the fourth ventricle may be stimulated by different chemicals and neurotransmitters as well as certain drugs.

Drugs that prevent vomiting work in many different ways.

DRUG	MECHANISM OF ACTION	SOME SIDE EFFECTS
Metoclopramide	Dopamine receptor antagonist	Movement disorders
	Increases gastric emptying	
Prochlorperazine Domperidone	Dopamine receptor antagonist	Drowsiness Movement disorders

DRUG	MECHANISM OF ACTION	SOME SIDE EFFECTS
Hyoscine	Acetylcholine receptor antagonist Action on vestibular apparatus in inner ear	Dry mouth and blurred vision Reduces gastric motility
Ondansetron	5-HT receptor antagonist	Flushing, hiccups
Cyclizine	Antihistamine	Drowsiness
Dexamethasone	Steroid. Reduces inflammatory mediators	Those of steroids

CAUSE OF VOMITING	EFFECTIVE DRUG CATEGORY
Chemotherapy – drugs with low risk of vomiting – prevention	Phenothiazines, e.g. **prochlorperazine** – may cause drowsiness. **Domperidone** may be used – less drowsiness Continue for 24 hours after treatment finishes
Chemotherapy drugs with a higher risk of vomiting	Add corticosteroid, e.g. **dexamethasone**, alone or with a benzodiazepine, e.g. **lorazepam**, prior to commencing therapy
Chemotherapy drugs with high risk	5-HT$_3$ antagonists, e.g. **ondansetron**. Usually effective

CAUSE OF VOMITING	EFFECTIVE DRUG CATEGORY
Post-surgery	***Prochlorperazine*** or ***metoclopramide*** (less effective). 5-HT$_3$ antagonists, e.g. ***ondansetron***, if necessary. Antihistamines, e.g. ***cyclizine***, may be used
Vomiting associated with GI tract, biliary or hepatic disease	***Metoclopramide*** may be more effective
Vomiting due to opioids	***Prochlorperazine, metoclopramide, cyclizine***
Migraine	***Metoclopramide, domperidone, phenothiazines*** or antihistamines may be used
Motion sickness	Should be given for prevention rather than treatment ***Hyoscine*** – transdermal patch applied a few hours before journey ***Cyclizine*** or ***cinnarizine*** (antihistamines) are also effective and may be better tolerated but cause drowsiness
Severe vomiting in pregnancy	Only rarely needed in first trimester – antihistamine, e.g. ***promethazine***

Analgesics

Drugs given for the relief of pain.

The analgesic ladder
Forms the basis of many approaches to the use of analgesic drugs.

There are essentially three steps:

1. **Non-opioids**, e.g. *paracetamol*, NSAIDs, e.g. *ibuprofen* – ceiling doses limit effects.
2. **Mild opioids**, e.g. *codeine*, *dihydrocodeine*. May be combined with paracetamol or a NSAID.
3. **Strong opioids** – e.g. *morphine*. Larger doses give greater pain relief with no ceiling effect.

Other drugs used for pain relief include local anaesthetics, centrally acting non-opioid drugs such as some antidepressants, e.g. *amitriptyline*, and drugs for specific conditions, e.g. *carbamazepine* for trigeminal neuralgia, *ergotamine* for migraine.

Opioids produce analgesia by acting on the CNS. **Local anaesthetics** act peripherally and **NSAIDs** have both peripheral and central effects.

■ PARACETAMOL

- Most frequently used analgesic for mild to moderate pain.
- Also used in pyrexia to decrease body temperature.
- Does not have anti-inflammatory action.
- Mechanism of action still not fully understood – now believed to stimulate cannabinoid receptors.

- Few side effects and safe in the elderly but toxic to liver cells if normal dose exceeded.
- Adult dose: 1 g (two tablets) every 4–6 hours with maximum of 4 g in 24 hours.

■ NSDAIDS

e.g. *aspirin, ibuprofen, naproxen, fenbufen, diclofenac, piroxicam*
- Very useful in chronic inflammatory conditions, e.g. arthritis.
- Pain relief is immediate but full anti-inflammatory action takes up to three weeks.
- All work by inhibiting the enzyme cyclo-oxygenase (COX) needed for the synthesis of prostaglandins.
- Side effect of gastritis and peptic ulcer formation due to thin mucosal lining in gut. Frequently presents as haematemesis, especially in the elderly. May limit their use.
- Newer selective COX-2 inhibitors, e.g. *celecoxib, etoricoxib, lumiracoxib*, do not have gastric side effects but increased incidence of myocardial infarction so not used in those at high risk of CVD.
- *Aspirin* used in small doses (75 mg daily) as antiplatelet drug in CVD prevention.
- NSAIDs should not to be given to asthmatics as some are aspirin-sensitive.

■ OPIOIDS

Used to relieve moderate to severe pain, especially if visceral. Powerful analgesics and change the perception of pain.

Tolerance and **dependence** may occur with repeated administration.

Most used is *morphine* derived from the opium poppy. Also produces euphoria and a sense of detachment from surroundings.

All are agonists at the opioid receptors in the CNS.

One major side effect in large doses is **respiratory depression**.

Other side effects include nausea, vomiting, constipation and drowsiness.

Pinpoint pupils are a sign that opioids have been taken.

Antidote to all opioids is *naloxone* – an opioid antagonist. It has a shorter life than morphine and so in cases of overdose will need to be repeated or given by continuous infusion.

■ SOME COMMON OPIOIDS

DRUG	DESCRIPTION
Morphine	Standard opioid and powerful analgesic to which all other opioids are compared.
Diamorphine (heroin)	Powerful. Enters brain readily. Used in palliative care. Popular with addicts
Fentanil Alfentanil Remifentanil	Very potent. Used during operations as analgesia. Fentanil also available as patches and lozenges that are used in palliative care.

DRUG	DESCRIPTION
Meptazinol	Claimed to have less respiratory depressant action.
Methadone	Longer acting and less sedating. Used as pain relief and in drug dependency when weaning off heroin.
Oxycodone	Control of pain in palliative care. Available as suppositories.
Pethidine	Less constipating but less potent.
Tramadol	Also acts on serotonin and adrenaline pathways. Less constipation and respiratory depression. Used in tablet form for moderate to severe pain.
Codeine	Too constipating for long-term use but effective for moderate pain.
Dihydrocodeine	Similar to codeine in analgesic effect.
Buprenorphine	Agonist and antagonist at opioid receptors. Only partially reversed by naloxone. Longer acting than morphine and available sublingually (acts for 6–8 hours). Can produce withdrawal symptoms in addicts. Is dependency-producing itself.

Drugs to treat diabetes mellitus

■ DIFFERENT ACTIONS OF VARIOUS TYPES OF INSULIN

TYPES OF INSULIN	BRAND NAMES	DESCRIPTION	FOLLOWING SUBCUTANEOUS ADMINISTRATION		
			ONSET	PEAK	DURATION
Quick-acting insulin					
Recombinant human insulin analogues	Insulin Lispro (*Humalog*) Insulin Aspart (*NovoRapid*) Insulin Glulisine (*Apidra*)	Amino acid structure slightly altered to make action faster and of shorter duration	5–20 min	30–60 min	2–5 hours 2–4 hours
Soluble insulin (insulin injection; neutral insulin)	Human sequence insulins: *Actrapid, Humulin S, Velosulin, Insuman Rapid* Highly purified animal insulins: *Hypurin Bovine Neutral Hypurin Porcine Neutral Pork Actrapid*	Structure as in the human body Porcine 1 AA different to human	30–60 min	2–4 hours	4–8 hours

Intermediate-acting insulins

Types of insulin	Brand names	Description			
Isophane insulin (Isophane protamine, Isophane NPH)	Insulatard, Humulin I, Insuman Basal *Porcine and Bovine Isophane, Pork Insulatard*	Soluble insulin and the protein protamine in equal amounts	1–2 hours	5–8 hours	12–18 hours

Long-acting insulins

Types of insulin	Brand names	Description			
Insulin zinc suspension	*Hipurin Bovine Lente Hipurin Bovine PZI*	Combined with zinc for longer action	1–2 hours	6–20 hours	Up to 36 hours
Basal insulin analogue	Glargine (Lantus) Detemir (Levemir)	Amino acid structure changed – long action for basal level	90 min	Flat profile	24 hours

TYPES OF INSULIN	BRAND NAMES	DESCRIPTION
Biphasic insulins		
Biphasic Insulin Aspart	*NovoMix 30*	Mixture of 30% fast-acting aspart and 70% intermediate-acting aspart protamine
Biphasic Insulin Lispro	*Humalog Mix 25 Humalog Mix 50*	25% or 50% fast-acting insulin lispro and 75% or 50% intermediate-acting insulin lispro protamine

■ ORAL HYPOGLYCAEMIC AGENTS AND THEIR ACTION

TYPE OF DRUG	NAME	MODE OF ACTION	SPECIAL FEATURES	SIDE EFFECTS
Sulphonylureas	*Gliclazide* *Glibenclamide* *Tolbutamide* *Glipizide*	Augment insulin secretion Need residual pancreatic activity	May rarely cause hypoglycaemia (hypo) – especially in elderly – may last many hours – treat in hospital Can encourage weight gain	Usually mild and infrequent Gastrointestinal, e.g. nausea, diarrhoea, constipation
Biguanides	*Metformin*	Decreases gluconeogenesis Increases peripheral utilisation of glucose	Drug of choice in Type 2 Do not gain weight Very little danger of hypo Reduced risk of CVD	Anorexia, nausea, diarrhoea, metallic taste, lactic acidosis

TYPE OF DRUG	NAME	MODE OF ACTION	SPECIAL FEATURES	SIDE EFFECTS
Glitazones	*Pioglitazone* *Rosiglitazone*	Reduce peripheral insulin resistance	Used with other oral hypoglycaemics Not with insulin	Check liver function tests Higher incidence of fractures in females
Meglitinides	*Repaglinide* *Nateglinide*	Stimulate insulin release	Rapid onset, short duration of action	Hypoglycaemia Rashes
Glucosidase inhibitor	*Acarbose*	Enzyme inhibitor – delays digestion of starch and sucrose	May be used in combination with oral drugs or insulin	Flatulence, soft stools, diarrhoea
DPP-4 inhibitor	*Sitagliptin* *Vildagliptin* *Saxagliptin*	Inhibits enzyme DPP-4. Slows inactivation of incretin hormones	May be used in combination with sulphonylurea or metformin. Not with insulin	Allergic reactions, runny nose, sore throat, headache
Incretin mimetic	*Exenatide* *Liraglutide*	Stimulates insulin secretion when glucose levels raised	In combination with metformin/ sulphonylureas if not controlled on max doses	Nausea, vomiting Hypoglycaemia

Some antibacterial drugs

DRUG GROUPS	FEATURES AND USES	UNWANTED EFFECTS
Penicillins Ampicillin, amoxicillin, azlocillin, benzylpenicillin (Penicillin G), Co-amoxiclav, flucloxacillin, phenoxymethylpenicillin (Penicillin V), piperacillin, Pivampicillin, ticarcillin	Beta-lactam antibiotic. Kills bacteria by interfering with cell wall synthesis. Most commonly prescribed and used for many infections Some bacteria have developed resistance, especially staphylococci	Very safe. High therapeutic index. Diarrhoea may occur. Allergy is main danger. Hypersensitivity causes rashes and anaphylaxis. Can be fatal
Cephalosporins Cefotazime, ceftazidime, cefuroxime, cefalexin, cefradine	Beta-lactam. Work in a similar way to penicillin. Broad spectrum. Used for septicaemia, pneumonia, meningitis, peritonitis, UTIs	Main danger is allergy as with penicillin

DRUG GROUPS	FEATURES AND USES	UNWANTED EFFECTS
Carbapenems Imipenem, meropenem, etrapenem	Broad spectrum. Work in similar way to other beta-lactams	Main side effect is allergy
Tetracyclines Tetracycline, doxycycline, lymecycline, minocycline	Broad spectrum. Used less now due to resistance. Used for chlamydia infections	GI upset. Antacids and milk prevent absorption
Tigecycline	Related to tetracyclines. Effective against MRSA and vancomycin resistant enterococci.	Reserved for complicated infections.

DRUG GROUPS	FEATURES AND USES	UNWANTED EFFECTS
Aminoglycosides Gentamicin, amikacin, netilmicin, tolramycin, neomycin	Bacteriocidal. Not absorbed from gut. Given IV unless for bowel. Used in severe infections, e.g. septicaemia	Dose-related deafness and renal damage. Levels in serum monitored
Macrolides Erythromycin (also azithromycin and clarithromycin)	Erythromycin has similar spectrum of action to penicillin. Used in penicillin sensitive and RTIs	Erythromycin irritant to GI tract – nausea, vomiting, diarrhoea. Rashes
Vancomycin, teicoplanin	Active against MRSA and treats *C. difficile*. Given IV	Kidney damage and blood disorders

The central nervous system

■ DRUGS COMMONLY USED TO PREVENT SEIZURES IN EPILEPSY

SEIZURE TYPE	FIRST LINE DRUGS
Tonic-clonic (grand mal)	Carbamazepine Lamotrigine Sodium valproate Topiramate
Absence (petit mal)	Ethosuximide Sodium valproate
	Lamotrigine
Myoclonic	Sodium valproate
Atonic	Lamotrigine
	Sodium Valproate

■ PARKINSON'S DISEASE

Due to a lack of the neurotransmitter dopamine in certain areas of the brain concerned with movement.

Drugs used to treat may:

- Be a precursor of dopamine (*levodopa*)
- Prevent destruction of dopamine (*selegiline*)
- Be a dopamine agonist (e.g. *bromocriptine*)
- Cause the release of dopamine (e.g. *amantidine*)

Co-beneldopa (Madopar®) is levodopa and bensarazide.
Co-careldopa (Sinemet®) is levodopa and carbidopa.

These combinations lessen some of the unwanted effects of dopamine outside the CNS.

■ ALZHEIMER'S DISEASE AND OTHER FORMS OF DEMENTIA

Donepezil, galantamine, rivastigmine

- Dementia may be due to a lack of acetylcholine in certain areas of the brain.
- Drugs are anticholinesterases that increase the activity of acetylcholine by inhibiting the enzyme that destroys it.
- All are absorbed from the GI tract and can be given orally.
- They may cause nausea and vomiting, diarrhoea and abdominal pain.
- In some patients they may cause insomnia and confusion.
- Prescribed by specialists in the treatment of dementia.

Antidepressants

Note that antidepressants do not work fully for several weeks. It is dangerous to prescribe more than one type of drug at once and often one drug must be withdrawn for a period before another drug is started (see BNF). Drugs should be withdrawn slowly if possible.

CLASS AND EXAMPLES	MODE OF ACTION	USES	UNWANTED EFFECTS
Tricyclics (TCAs) Amitriptyline, clomipramine, dosulepin (dothiepin), doxepin, imipramine, lofepramine	Prevent reuptake of noradrenaline and serotonin into the nerve cell and so prolong action at synapse. Also anticholinergic	Moderate to severe depression. Often aid sleeping. Useful in neuropathic pain	Arrhythmias. Drowsiness. Anticholinergic – dry mouth, blurred vision, constipation, retention of urine. Sweating. May be fatal in overdose – arrhythmias, convulsions, coma and respiratory depression
MAOIs Phenelzine, moclobemide (reversible)	Block the enzyme that destroys amines such as noradrenaline	Depression that does not respond to other drugs. Used less because of interactions with food	Interact with certain foods and drugs (see BNF). Moclobemide less. Many of same side effects as TCAs. Dangerous in overdose

CLASS AND EXAMPLES	MODE OF ACTION	USES	UNWANTED EFFECTS
SSRIs Citalopram, escitalopram, fluoxetine, paroxetine, sertraline	Block the reuptake of serotonin and so raise serotonin levels in the CNS	Depression. Anxiety states. Bulimia nervosa. Obsessive-compulsive disorder, panic disorder. Post-traumatic stress disorder	Less dangerous in overdose. Not so toxic to the heart. Fewer side effects. Do not cause drowsiness – may cause insomnia, anorexia and weight loss. Some may increase suicide risk in the young. Serotonin syndrome

Other drugs that work by different mechanisms and are used by specialists include *mirtazapine*, *reboxetine* and *venlafaxine*.

Hypnotics

Drugs to aid sleeping.
- Only used for short periods when absolutely necessary.
- May be habit forming.
- Benzodiazepines (BZs), e.g. *nitrazepam, flurazepam, temazepam, loprazolam*.
- Newer drugs that are not BZs but do act as BZ receptor include *zaleplon, zolpidem* and *zopiclone*. Have a short duration of action but dependence has been reported.

Antipsychotic drugs

- Also known as neuroleptics and major tranquillisers.
- Used in mental health to treat schizophrenia.
- Occasionally used to treat severe anxiety.
- All block types of dopamine receptor in the brain and have extrapyramidal side effects associated with this and leading to movement disorders (Parkinsonian side effects). Atypical drugs have fewer unwanted effects.
- Drugs include *chlorpromazine, haloperidol, pipotiazine, fluphenazine* and *flupentixol.*
- Newer atypical drugs include *clozapine, risperidone, quetiapine* and *olanzapine.*
- Drugs are sometimes given as depot injections.

Mania – the main drug used to treat is *lithium*.

Adverse drug reactions

An adverse drug reaction (ADR) is an unwanted or unintended effect of medicine that occurs during proper use.

No drug is administered without some risk.

New ADRs should be reported using the yellow card found at the back of the BNF.

Divided into Type A and Type B reactions:

TYPE A ADVERSE DRUG REACTIONS (AUGMENTED)	TYPE B ADVERSE DRUG REACTIONS (BIZARRE)
Predictable	Unpredictable
Related to the expected effects of the drug	Unrelated to the expected effects – may be due to allergic response
Dose dependent	Not dose dependent
Occur frequently	Rare
Low mortality	High mortality
Reduce drug dose if occur	Stop drug if occur
Less likely to result in withdrawal from market	May result in withdrawal of drug from market
Example is headache following GTN	Example is anaphylaxis following penicillin

■ PREDISPOSING FACTORS

- Polypharmacy (multiple drug therapy).
- Age – very old and very young.
- Gender – women appear more susceptible.
- Presence of other diseases such as HIV, cardiac disease, liver disease, kidney disease.

- Race – ethnic differences in drug handling.
- Hereditary differences in drug metabolising enzymes.

■ EXAMPLES OF ADRS

- **Skin reactions** – most commonly a rash – may be allergic in nature and subsequent exposure may lead to more severe effects such as anaphylaxis.
- **Gastrointestinal** – nausea and vomiting, loss of appetite, diarrhoea, constipation, gastritis.
- **Hepatic toxicity** – may depend on dose of drug, e.g. paracetamol. May need to monitor liver function, e.g. statins.
- **Blood disorders** – rare but serious, e.g. aplastic anaemia where RBCs, WBCs and platelets are reduced.
- **Cardiovascular** – may be predictable, e.g. postural hypotension with some antihypertensives.
- **Arrhythmias** – increased awareness that some drugs may cause cardiac arrhythmias and even sudden death in susceptible patients.

Adverse drug events

An adverse drug event (ADE) is actual or potential damage resulting from medical intervention related to medicines.

This definition could include ADRs but ADE is a term that is most frequently used in association with medication errors.

Medication errors are preventable events that may cause or lead to patient harm. Medication errors are always avoidable whereas some ADRs are unpredictable and therefore unavoidable. It is important to distinguish between an ADR and a medication error when ADEs are reported.

Medication errors usually occur when human error or system failure interact with the prescribing, dispensing or administration of drugs with an unintended and potentially harmful outcome.

■ SOME PRESCRIBING AND ADMINISTRATION ERRORS

- Incorrect selection of the drug.
- Incorrect dose or frequency of administration.
- Incorrect route of administration.
- Wrong length of therapy.
- Prescribing or administering drugs that interact.
- Prescribing or administering drugs that the patient has a known allergy to.
- Illegible prescription.
- Incorrect patient given the drug.

■ POSSIBLE CAUSES OF PRESCRIBING AND ADMINISTRATION ERRORS

- Insufficient knowledge of the patient and their illness.
- Poor history taking, e.g. allergy identification.
- Inadequate knowledge of the drug prescribed.
- Calculation errors of drug dose.
- Illegible handwriting.
- Inadequate checking of patient identity and drug dose.
- Inadequate drug monitoring.
- Medicine administered but not taken by the patient.

ADE reporting must be encouraged even when the patient is not likely to be harmed by the error. Although the error may appear to be a human error, it is most often the system that is at fault. To design safer systems, errors must be reported and all possible contributory factors should be looked at and analysed. There may be an identifiable chain of events that have led to the error.

■ PREVENTING ERRORS

- Readily available information about all aspects of drugs prescribed.
- Good education of all members of the healthcare team involved in prescribing and administering of drugs.
- Accessible information about the patient, their condition and any allergies.
- Good history taking and documentation.
- Avoidance of excessive workloads that may lead to errors and memory lapses.
- Avoiding illegibility – all drug names should be printed in UPPER CASE letters and only acceptable abbreviations should be used.
- Careful use of zeros and decimal points. 'Trailing' zeros should never be used, e.g. 1.0 mg as this can be mistaken for 10 mg – should always be written 1 mg. Leading zeros should always be used, e.g. 0.1 mg and not .1 mg.
- Encouragement of a 'no blame' culture and ensuring staff feel comfortable to ask questions and report errors.
- Good communication.
- Careful drug monitoring.
- Checking medication dose and route with another staff member.
- Awareness of high risk areas of practice, e.g. calculation errors occur most frequently in paediatrics where there are wide variations in dose according to body weight.

- The BNF gives guidance on prescription writing and all drugs – an up-to-date copy should always be available for referral.
- Treatment plans should include monitoring for both therapeutic and unwanted effects of drugs.
- Drug treatment should be discussed with the patient if at all possible.

Drug and food interactions

Food may interact with drugs in several ways, as described below.

Absorption from the gastrointestinal tract

- Rate of absorption – not usually important unless immediate action is needed, e.g. pain relief. Fluids may increase the rate of absorption and solid, heavy meals decrease the rate.
- Extent of absorption. This is decreased by food if drugs are not lipid soluble, e.g. *atenolol*.
- Gastric acid and enzymes may destroy some drugs, e.g. *penicillin*.
- Some drugs are chelated by certain metal ions, e.g. *tetracycline* by calcium (in milk) or iron. If the drug is taken with these substances it will not be absorbed.

Distribution around the body

An example is a high protein diet decreasing the level of the anti-Parkinson drug *levodopa*. This is because amino acids compete with the transport of levodopa across the blood–brain barrier.

Metabolism and clearance of the drug

Certain foods stimulate liver enzymes that metabolise drugs. This means the drug level in the body is decreased. Examples include:

- Barbecued foods.
- Broccoli, cabbage and Brussels sprouts.

Other substances may inhibit drug metabolising enzymes. For example:

- Grapefruit juice is an important example and increases the levels of many important drugs including statins and *amlodipine*.
- Cranberry juice inhibits the enzyme that metabolises *warfarin*.

Interaction with receptors or sites of drug action

Vitamin K competes with warfarin so foods high in Vitamin K, e.g. broccoli and leafy green vegetables, decrease the activity of *warfarin*.

Alcohol increases the sedatory effects of drugs acting on the CNS and may also increase any respiratory depressant effects of drugs such as opioids and benzodiazepines.

MAOI antidepressants may cause a hypertensive crisis when foods rich in tyramine such as marmite and strong cheeses are eaten.

Some differentiating features of drug overdose

■ DRUGS CAUSING COMA

Depress the CNS:
- hypnotics
- antidepressants
- anticonvulsants
- tranquillisers
- opioid analgesics
- alcohol

■ DRUGS AFFECTING PUPIL SIZE

CONSTRICTED PUPILS	DILATED PUPILS
Cholinergics	Amphetamines
Opiates	Anticholinergics, e.g. atropine
Physostigmine	Antihistamines
Phenothiazines	Cocaine
Valproate	LSD
	Tricyclic antidepressants

■ DRUGS CAUSING RESPIRATORY FEATURES

- Hypoventilation and respiratory depression common with CNS depressants. Marked rate reduction usually due to **opioids**.
- Hyperventilation may be due to **salicylate** poisoning, CNS stimulant drugs or cyanide.
- Pulmonary oedema with inhaled poisons or some herbicides, e.g. *paraquat*.

- Cough, wheeze and breathlessness – inhalation of irritant gases such as ammonia or chlorine and smoke from fires.
- Cyanosis due to a combination of factors in the unconscious patient or methaemoglobinaemia caused by poisons such as chlorates, nitrates, nitrites, phenol and urea herbicides.

■ CARDIOVASCULAR FEATURES

- **Tachycardia** with anticholinergics, sympathomimetics and salicylates.
- **Bradycardia** may be caused by *digoxin* and beta-blockers.
- **Arrhythmias** caused by many drugs especially tricyclic antidepressants, some antihistamines and some antipsychotics. Many antiarrhythmic drugs cause dysrhythmias if taken in excess.
- **Hypotension** may occur in any severe poisoning.
- **CNS depressants** may lower the systolic blood pressure.
- **Diuretics** lower the blood pressure by depleting the blood volume.
- **Hypertension** is uncommon in overdosage but may occur following sympathomimetics such as **amphetamines**.

BRADYCARDIA OR AV BLOCK	TACHYCARDIA
Beta-blockers	Amphetamines
Digoxin	Antihistamines
Dispyramide	Atropine
Flecainide	Caffeine
Opiates	Carbon monoxide
Organophosphates	Cocaine
Physostigmine	Theophylline
Tricyclics	Tricyclics
Rate-limiting calcium channel blockers	

Common drug overdoses

DRUG	DANGEROUS DOSE CAUSE OF DEATH	ANTIDOTE/TREATMENT	SIGNS AND SYMPTOMS
Paracetamol (Acetaminophen)	20–30 tablets Liver failure due to metabolite toxic to liver cells	Acetylcysteine (Parvolex) by infusion or oral methionine Activated charcoal Paracetamol level 4 hours after ingestion Treat according to graph in BNF	Delay of about 24 hours before symptom onset but liver enzymes raised after 12 hours. May have some nausea. Pain in right upper quadrant of abdomen Tenderness, nausea, vomiting and jaundice. Liver failure, cerebral oedema and death

DRUG	DANGEROUS DOSE CAUSE OF DEATH	ANTIDOTE/TREATMENT	SIGNS AND SYMPTOMS
Aspirin (Salicylate)	2 tablets/kg toxic Death may occur due to cardiovascular collapse, seizures and hyperthermia or pulmonary oedema	Activated charcoal No antidote Serum salicylate levels Monitor blood gases and electrolytes Alkalinise the urine to increase excretion. Haemodialysis	May begin in 1–2 hours, peaks 12–24 hours Tinnitus, vomiting, bleeding. Stimulates respiratory centre – hyperventilation and respiratory alkalosis Lactic acidosis Increased body temperature, tachycardia.
Tricyclic antidepressants	Less than 10 times the normal dose. Dangerous cardiac arrhythmias and seizures	Airway, breathing, circulation (ABC). ECG. Activated charcoal Treat seizures with diazepam Alkalisation increases binding and lowers levels	Anticholinergic first – dry mouth, life-threatening seizures Wide complex tachycardias, hypotension, coma May deteriorate rapidly

DRUG	DANGEROUS DOSE CAUSE OF DEATH	ANTIDOTE/TREATMENT	SIGNS AND SYMPTOMS
Beta-blockers	Differ in toxicity. 2–3 times normal dose is toxic in some Death due to cardiac arrest	Activated charcoal if OK Atropine to combat bradycardia and hypotension. ECG Glucagon 2–10 mg in Dextrose 5%. Inotropes. May need pacemaker	Some remain asymptomatic Bradycardia and hypotension Atrioventricular block, ventricular arrhythmias, cardiac arrest Sedation or coma. Occasionally seizures
Calcium channel blockers	Verapamil most dangerous. All need immediate attention. Very dangerous in children	ABC. Advanced life support if needed Activated charcoal if OK. IV calcium chloride or gluconate. Atropine for bradycardia. May treat hypotension with inotropes	Nausea, vomiting, dizziness, agitation, confusion, bradycardia, cardiogenic shock, hypotension, syncope, lethargy, coma, hyperglycaemia

Useful websites

----

www.resus.org.uk
Resuscitation Council (UK)

www.nice.org.uk
National Institute of Health and Clinical Excellence

www.bnf.org
British National Formulary online

www.homeoffice.gov.uk/drugs/
Home Office drug website

www.pharmweb.net
Pharmacy information for patients and professionals

www.healthcarerepublic.com/publications/MIMS
Electronic MIMS

www.nmc-uk.org
Nursing and Midwifery Council (UK)

www.dh.gov.uk
Department of Health

www.mhra.gov.uk
Medicines and Healthcare Products Regulation Agency

www.prescriber.co.uk
Prescriber journal website

Shift roster

DAY	DATE	SHIFT
MONDAY		
TUESDAY		
WEDNESDAY		
THURSDAY		
FRIDAY		
SATURDAY		
SUNDAY		